Elephants in Arkansas

THE MUSINGS OF AN ARKANSAS VETERINARIAN

Elephants in Arkansas
The Musings of an Arkansas Veterinarian

Available in eBook and Paperback

Print ISBN: 978-1733106412

NKB Books, LLC
Canyon, Texas

Editor: Natalie Bright
Cover Design: NKB Books, LLC
Cover Photo: Canva Pro

Dedicated to my father, Richard Keith Fulton.

He was a veterinarian for thirty-eight years. His practice included many separate types of veterinary medicine including small animals, large animals, and industrial.

He encouraged and inspired me in my career.

CHAPTER 1
ELEPHANTS IN ARKANSAS

AT FIRST THOUGHT, you might not consider central Arkansas being the home of one of the largest herds of both Asian and African elephants in the nation, but it's true. I also would have never dreamed that elephant medicine would become such a prominent part of my practice for a period of time.

One fall day in the late nineties a large trailer pulled up in the clinic's parking lot. A man introduced himself as Mr. Scott Riddle, and he came with an unusual request. He was hoping to find a local veterinarian to fill out and sign a health certificate so that he could transport a young elephant from Arkansas to Florida.

Completely surprised by his request, my curiosity and his obvious enthusiasm for these animals won me over. I was willing but wanted to call the state veterinarian's Board to find out what was required. After I had finished meeting with Scott, he asked If I would be interested in being the veterinarian for his elephant breeding center and sanctuary. I couldn't help but be fascinated by the idea, but I had concerns because I had no experience with these animals. Of all the places I've lived in my life, I can honestly say an elephant has never crossed my path.

After talking to Scott and learning more about his operation, I agreed to the challenge of the job, if he would get me in contact with some elephant experts. He more than exceeded my request when he introduced me to one of the Ringling Brothers veterinarians as well as one of the premier veterinary reproductive specialists in the country. This began a long-term relationship with Scott and his wife Heidi, and one that changed my practice for the better allowing me to work with these amazing and complicated animals.

There are so many great stories involving Riddle Elephant Sanctuary, but one of my favorites occurred soon after I was married to my beautiful wife Kathy. The week after we had returned from our honeymoon, I got a call from Scott asking me to examine an older male African elephant that was having difficulties. I asked Kathy if she wanted to go, and she quickly agreed.

The sanctuary was still in the process of being built and they had not completed the fencing yet around their outdoor area. As Scott and I discussed the sick African, we noticed two elephants standing about 200 yards away next to a wire fence. The two adults were pushing playfully against each other. Scott became concerned that they might push each other into the fence. I expected that he would quickly head in their direction, but what he did surprised me. He proved to me just how smart these huge animals really are.

The young male was named Booper, and Mary was a mature female. Scott yelled out a command, "Booper, forward. Mary, back."

To my complete amazement Booper took two steps forward and Mary took two steps back. The intelligence it takes to process and fulfill these commands is beyond that of most, if not all, animals that I know of. On top of that these magnificent beasts followed these instructions immediately, without hesitation, and at a very long distance. If I was not before, I was now and will forever be a fan of this amazing species.

A few minutes later another staff member brought Mary and Booper closer to a small enclosure next to the barn where they were kept at night. Kathy watched as these two tried to make their way into the barn where hay and grain was being put out for their nightly feeding. Scott was in the habit of keeping them out of the barn until all of the elephants had been brought up. As he and I continued our discussion on the patient, Kathy noticed that Mary and Booper were intent on sneaking into the barn. Whenever Scott's attention was diverted, both elephants would take a step or two closer to the barn. When Scott looked their way, he gently commanded them to step back. They would immediately do as asked, but then the minute he looked away they ducked their heads and took two more steps forward. Kathy could not help but laugh as this game continued. The only problem with their plan is that it's most difficult to "sneak" when you're a 6,000-pound elephant.

After this, I turned my attention back to my patient. I still needed to figure out what was wrong with Toby the African Male. Scott and I discussed the symptoms and the previous problems that Toby had been dealing with. We determined that he was in pain from swelling brought on by the worsening symptoms of arthritis. I assessed the need for anti-inflammatories and felt that he would show much improvement.

The problem was that the best way to administer medication to an elephant is to give them intravenously. There are two places commonly used to give IV's on elephants. One of the easiest areas is the veins in the large ears of African elephants. The second problem I faced with this procedure was the product I had prescribed could cause severe inflammation if it got outside of the vein. If this happened, it could cause the ear to become so badly affected that it could possibly fall off. This was a chance I could not take.

The decision was made to give the IV product through the second optimal site on the animal; the vein located on the inside of one of the rear legs. There was not as much danger in this location, if it got outside of the vein. As for my part, I'd be lying under this magnificent beast injecting a needle into the site. As I prepared to slide under Toby to give the meds and ease his discomfort, Scott quietly mentioned that I might want to be as quick as possible.

I glanced at my new bride and saw a look of concern on her face. I gathered all my equipment, took a deep breath, and moved into position under Toby's leg. The procedure went very quickly.

I shook hands with Scott, and we said our goodbyes. On the drive home, I asked Kathy if she enjoyed visiting the farm. She told me she had but related her fears of having a one-ton creature falling on her new husband. Kathy mentioned that she couldn't help but visualize the local newspaper headlines, *"Local Veterinarian's Wife Widowed by Falling Elephant"*.

We shared a nervous laugh, and then I told her I would do my best to keep that headline from ever happening.

Every time I worked with the elephants, I remembered the promise I had made to my new wife. I always felt safe being around these magnificent animals, but I also knew that I needed to take precautions. Scott and his crew definitely put my safety as a top priority, and during the many years I worked with them, I never felt like I was in any significant danger.

> *The most obvious distinguishing characteristic between the African and Asian elephant are the ears. African elephants have the large fan-shaped ears which are used to dissipate heat from their body. The ears on Asian elephants are smaller and rounder. African elephants are considered to be the largest land mammals on Earth.*

CHAPTER 2
GET UP YOU S.O.B.

EARLY IN MY veterinary career in Greenbrier Arkansas I lived in a 3-bedroom mobile home located just across the driveway from the clinic. As a single man it was the perfect setup: low-cost rent with a thirty second commute to work. The disadvantage was that clients thought it was no big deal to come over and knock on my door after hours for emergencies and non-emergencies alike.

Very early one Sunday morning I suddenly awoke from a deep and sound sleep. Looking at the clock beside my bed I noted that it was a very early 3:15 A.M.

Lying in bed wondering what had startled me so early I heard a banging noise outside my window. Opening the curtains just enough to see across the driveway, I noticed a truck and trailer backed up into the large animal area. Still sleepy, I quickly became very frustrated as well. It was an unspoken rule that clients would call me first if they had an emergency. I slowly rolled out of bed, found my pants on a nearby chair and sat back down on the bed to pull them on. I was grumbling to myself wondering how they would feel if I showed up at their house in the middle of the night. At exactly that moment I heard a man yell, his voice ringing clear in the stillness of the early morning. "Get up you son-of-a-bitch!"

My mood instantly changed from moderate frustration and sleepiness to complete and total anger. I do not get angry easily, but those aggressive words had flipped a switch in my brain and suddenly I was as mad as I could ever remember in a very long time. I jumped up off the bed and almost fell on my face as I tried to pull my pants on. With no shirt or shoes, I began a determined run-stumble through the trailer. All I remember is that I had made a sudden decision that I was about to be in a fight with no real consideration of the consequences. I was not taking this from anyone! As I passed through the kitchen, I looked out the window to see how big this dude was that I was about to take on. What I saw once again caused a sudden and complete change of mood from complete anger to laughter.

The man was not yelling obscenities at me as I had thought, but he had been desperately yelling at his horse to get up off the trailer floor. It was not my normal attitude to laugh at clients' desperation or patients' problems, but probably the relief in the fact that I was not about to find myself in a fist fight with a client had caused my crazy change in attitude once again.

I quickly went back to my bedroom and finished dressing. As I left the trailer I was still laughing, and I noticed that my client was looking at me with some confusion. I suspect he was wondering if I was drunk or crazy to be laughing after being routed out of my bed this early in the morning. I immediately started the process of helping him get his bay stallion named Buck off the floor of the trailer and into the clinic.

The stallion was able to get up and out of the trailer without a great deal of difficulty, but then he immediately tried to lie back down. His eyes were wide open as if in a state of panic. Buck's breathing rate was increased, and he just could not seem to get comfortable. I first was able to reduce his discomfort by giving him an intravenous pain medication. His breathing rate returned to normal, and he was able to stand comfortably. After doing a full exam including listening to his abdomen with a stethoscope, I was able to diagnose a serious case of intestinal blockage and pain called colic. Buck's problem was most likely due to his habit of stealing more than his share of grain from the other horses in the pasture. This had resulted in a blockage of his small intestine which then caused serious pain. Any intestinal pain in horses can be very intense and will cause them to thrash around and can even lead to fatal conditions such as twisted intestine.

We ran Buck into a chute. Quickly gathering the supplies I needed, I performed a procedure in which a tube is placed through the nose of the horse. A gallon of mineral oil is pumped through the tube and into the stomach. This is the only way to give the needed volume of the oil into the intestine of the horse. With the pain meds in effect Buck did not resist this procedure and quickly the lubricant oil was where it needed to be. Thankfully in this case the pain meds as well as the mineral oil was able to relieve the intestinal impaction and the colic pain that it caused. Within three hours of his arrival, I was able to send a comfortable Buck and a relieved owner back home.

About two weeks later I happened to see this same client at the local coffee shop. He was a former bull rider, much smaller in stature than me, but the scars on his arms and face proved he wasn't one to run from a scrap. After inquiring about Buck and finding out that his horse had recovered well with no further complications, I asked if I could join him for a minute. He nodded his head and invited me to sit down. I proceeded to tell him my explanation of how his yelling got me riled up and ready for a fight until I had realized the truth. He quietly listened to me as I talked with a blank expression on his face.

After I finished, he took a sip of his coffee, looked at me with a wry smile, and replied, “It would have been hell to have to whoop the vet at 3 o’clock in the morning.”

CHAPTER 3
YOU SNEAK-EM BUFFALO

IT WAS a cold early spring morning as I climbed into my clinic truck to head out for this unusual emergency call. I had received a call from Nancy Simpson earlier that morning imploring me to come out to her farm to help save her Bison cow, commonly called Buffalo, that had been in labor for over 24 hours. She felt her prize cow was suffering and she was basically begging me to do something.

As I drove out, I recalled the events that had brought us to this point. Nancy and her husband Ed owned a very progressive farm twelve miles out of town.

They were in year four of an ambitious project to raise and breed buffalo for resale as well as for meat production. From the beginning they had planned well and had bought the best equipment so that they could make their dream farm a reality.

Raising buffalo is not easy and has several issues that make it much more difficult than having a cow-calf operation. Heat and humidity found in the south is not the natural habitat where most American buffalo inhabited. The Simpsons had provided barns and cover to help them deal with the Arkansas spa-like temperatures in the summer. The other factor that makes them difficult to raise is that they are hard to keep contained in normal fences that would work for cattle. A great deal of time and money had been spent building adequate fencing to keep these powerful animals inside the enclosures. Bulls can weigh up to 2000 lbs. and be up to 6 feet tall. Over 75% of their weight and power is in the front legs, shoulders, neck, and head. By comparison the rear quarters are much lighter and less powerful. This means that facilities used to handle cattle do not work well for buffaloes.

The Simpsons had built a special set of pens and chutes that could be used for working the calves and yearlings. Unfortunately, no matter how big or strong you built the chutes they did not work well on the adults. The adult cows and bulls would get over-excited and would run full speed into the pens and chutes. This would do serious damage to the property, but more importantly could severely injure the animals.

Early in the planning and developing of a herd health program we had made the decision that we would not attempt to run the adults through the chute system. I had made it clear that this meant that if any of the cows had difficulty calving, we would not be able to get them up to pull the calf. We learned from other producers that it was best to not try to treat these cows. Most cows would survive although the calf would not.

I had been called out to see the cow the afternoon before. I had reminded Nancy about our earlier agreement to not try to corral the expectant mother. She had reluctantly agreed with me, and I left the farm with the cow still in labor. By the next morning the cow was in more pain and discomfort and Nancy was in tears. This policy of wait and see sounded fine till she was watching her "babies" suffer.

The Simpsons had already tried earlier in the morning to push the mother up into a set of pens. As soon as the cow had been isolated from its herd-mates it had begun to slam into the fences. They had abandoned that idea. It was at this point when I had been called out again to the farm.

After looking at all possible options I could see only two viable ways to go. We could just watch the mother for the next few days to weeks to see if she would survive or we could try to sedate the mother with anesthetic darts. I cautioned them that there were no guarantees and that there was a possibility that the anesthetic could kill the mother. As soon as I mentioned the anesthetic option Nancy was dead set on that course of action.

I contacted a friend of mine that had a nearby vet practice who had bought a dart gun a few years previously. I had hoped that he would be able to come out to sedate the distressed buffalo for me. Unfortunately, he was busy with his own practice and the best he could do was let me use the dart gun. I had never used one before but was willing to give it a try. I sent an employee to borrow the dart gun, and I went back to the clinic to pick up the needed anesthetic.

As I prepared to do this, I was haunted by the possibility that this could turn into a major disaster. Who did I think I was, Marlin Perkins from Mutual of Omaha's *Wild Kingdom*? I took a deep breath and tried to eliminate the negative thoughts. They were not going to help anyone especially not Nancy and her "baby."

I gathered the needed anesthetic and loaded the darts. Hopping up into the back of Ed's truck, we entered the pen where the herd was located. We were able to get close to the cow, but I still managed to miss my first shot. I blamed it on a nasty north wind. My second dart found its target in the hind limb of the cow. Now it was just time to wait and watch the cow for the anesthetic to take effect.

Twenty minutes later the cow was showing very little sedation. I was cautious about giving too much anesthetic at one time, but it was obvious that I was going to need to increase the dose. Another dart was loaded, and we tracked her down, but she was now leery of the truck and once again it took two darts to successfully administer the dose. I could not believe that this also did not sufficiently sedate our patient. I only had one dart left so I felt pressure as we loaded a higher dose. Ed steered his truck toward the herd, and we headed out to try again. This time I was able to hit home on the first try. I had given enough sedative to put to sleep a regular cow three times her size. Now we waited to see if this high dose would finally work.

After fifteen minutes the buffalo cow finally lay down in a small grove of trees. As we approached, I was completely shocked when once again she rose and stumbled a few feet before falling. These animals were very powerful and unpredictable in this state and there was no way that I could try to pull the calf without more sedation. What was I to do now?

The only option was to give another dose of sedative, but I was out of darts. I was not happy about it, but the only idea I could come up with was to try to sneak up on her and quickly give her an intramuscular injection by syringe. I could not believe I was about to try this. I really was risking my own safety now. I took a deep breath, loaded the syringe, and slowly started moving toward the cow. As long as I walked slowly and remained quiet, she appeared to be agitated and did not try to move. I was carefully moving forward when I had a very strange thought.

The whole process of sneaking up on a buffalo made me think of a young Caddo brave doing the same a hundred years earlier with a knife in his hand instead of a syringe. The hunter may have garnered a name for his bravery and for efforts to provide meat for his family. Maybe I would earn such a name. How about "You Sneak-um Buffalo."

I shook myself out of my crazy daydreams and continued to move forward. I would use a tree as a protective barrier between myself and the cow after I gave the injection. Within seconds I stuck the plunger into her tough hide, administered the medication, and quickly moved away. She jumped a bit afterward but did not try to come after me. Within ten minutes she appeared to be soundly asleep, and I gathered my calf pulling equipment.

As I attempted to place a rope around her rear legs, she gave me a reminder that she was still a threat. Before I even knew she could move she kicked me twice in my upper leg. Thankfully the anesthetic reduced her power enough not to hurt me. I would have a good bruise to remind me of our encounter.

Ed helped secure his cow, then I

started the process of pulling the calf. Thankfully I was able to turn the head forward and placed light chains on both front feet. After spreading some lubricant around the calf, we started gentle but firm traction on the chains attached to the little hooves appearing in the birth canal. Five minutes of hard work and suddenly the calf began to be delivered. A bit more lubricant added and the calf slipped out of the cow. Unfortunately, it was quickly evident that the calf had been dead for some time. We knew from the start that the chance of a live calf was unlikely at best, but it was still heartbreaking. The goal at this point was to finish the process and save the mother.

I was able to place some antibiotic powder deep into the uterus and give a long-acting antibiotic injection. I felt this should help reduce the chance of any serious infection developing. Ed found a couple bales of hay nearby and as we removed the ropes on her legs, we carefully rolled her up onto her chest and propped her up with the bales. This should support her well until the anesthetic wore off and she was able to stand on her own.

I was still worried about the massive amount of anesthetic she had received but was pleasantly surprised when after fifteen minutes she was already trying to move her head about. We decided that it was time for us to move away from her and let her wake up slowly so that she would not hurt herself by trying to rise too quickly.

We set up just outside the fence where we could monitor her without providing any undo stimulation. Only then did the relief from the stress of the past several hours hit me. I knew that it would take at least the rest of the day for our patient to fully wake up, but as we watched her, I was feeling more and more confident that we had saved their precious 'Buffalo'. I gathered my equipment and limped back to my truck.

Nancy ran up to me and with tears in her eyes, gave me a big hug, and thanked me over and over again. These were counted as the moments that reminded me why I loved my job so much. As I pulled away from the farm, I smiled and remembered my self-given Native American name. Maybe I should just keep that to myself.

> “*The American Bison provided everything a Plains Indian family needed to survive the harsh environment of the North American pasture lands. This animal became the center of Tribal culture. Besides meat, thick hair became soft bedding and teepee shelter, and their bones were shaped into tools. Despite their impressive size, they can run up to 35 miles per hour.*

CHAPTER 4
GET OUT OF MY WAY, DOC

THE TERM USED when cows are having difficulty having a calf is called dystocia. This issue always seemed to happen more often than not late at night or when the weather was very bad. Every once in a while though, I would get a dystocia call during office hours. One of those calls occurred mid-morning on a beautiful spring day. Usually, I would drive out to the country to see my patients, but this time the pregnant cow was in a small tree-lined pasture within Greenbrier city limits.

Larry Johnson was the owner of the

small Angus cow that had been in labor all morning with no success to this point. As I rolled to a stop, I could see that he had placed the cow in a small pen next to the larger pasture. Larry was a middle-aged man who owned a modest cow herd as a second job. He built houses and managed a few apartment complexes as his main method of income. Although not a full-time farmer he had a good deal of experience with cattle and had a nice herd. I thanked him for having the cow caught up and ready for examination. I removed my calf pulling gear from my truck hoping for a quick, successful delivery.

The cow was lying on her side and pushing hard, but no parts of the calf could be seen. I put on a full arm length glove on my left arm and began my examination. The first thing I noticed was that the calf had not yet entered the pelvic canal. This was unusual because normally I would feel the head or at least one foot.

Finally, I was able to feel a very large calf deep in the uterus. It was immediately obvious that this calf was way too big to be born normally from this small cow. The good news was that I could feel strong movement of the calf as I felt around its head and front feet. It was then that I felt a sensation that did not happen often, but when it did it always thrilled me.

As I moved my hand around the head and mouth the unborn calf still in the womb began to suckle my gloved finger. I am sure this was just a reflex ingrained in the calf, but to me it always felt more like a miracle. It was now time to see if we could get this calf born alive so it could suckle for real. A C-section was the only way we were going to have a successful birth today. My hopes of a quick and easy delivery had evaporated. This would be a complicated and tedious procedure.

I explained the situation to Mr. Johnson and after only a brief moment of hesitation he gave me permission to go forward with the C-section. The cow would only stand for a moment or two before laying back down and continuing her labor pains. I made the decision to do the surgery with the cow lying on her side in this small pen. We placed a halter on her head and ropes around her front and rear legs to keep her from standing up in the middle of the procedure. It was too dangerous for both the cow and her calf to fully anesthetize her for a C-section, so I made the decision to do a local anesthetic block along the area of the abdomen where I would make the incision. This was the best way to provide a safe delivery and at the same time eliminate pain for the mother. Out in the field the only help I would have was that of the owner. For this reason, I had learned to prepare as thoroughly as possible and try to anticipate likely issues that might occur.

The next 30 minutes or so were spent

getting my surgical equipment ready. I explained the procedure to make sure that Larry could handle the position of surgical assistant. I could call for some help, but that would delay the surgery and possibly the success of getting a live calf. He gave me a big smile and told me he was up for the job. I then started the process of cleaning the skin and placing the local anesthetic under the skin. A C-section involves cutting through the skin, sub-cutaneous tissue, layers of muscle, and then through the uterus to the calf. After all these incisions are made the calf has to be physically removed from the abdomen of the cow. This is not a small job since the calf was over 90 lbs. in this case.

Larry did a great job assisting me to save this little bull calf. I quickly made sure that the calf was breathing then turned over the care of the newest herd member to my capable assistant. Larry was an experienced cowman, and he knew the process of making sure it was doing well. He first cleaned the afterbirth away from the nose and mouth so the bull could breathe with no obstructions. Next the naval cord was trimmed and a small amount of tincture of iodine was applied to the area to prevent infection. Larry gently laid the solid black calf on a soft bed of fresh hay. There he could breathe, gain some strength, and rest from his traumatic entrance into this new world.

The next reality in C-sections is that it takes a great deal less time to cut open the tissues to reach the calf than it does to sew it all back together. It took me less than 20 minutes to get the calf out, but the closure would take me over 45 minutes. I had closed the uterus and muscle and subcutaneous tissue, and deep in concentration, I focused on the process of closing the skin.

Suddenly I was shocked from my task by a bump in the middle of my back. I ignored it at first, assuming that Larry had maybe stumbled or accidentally fallen into me. A couple seconds later, I was hit again with a persistent push between my shoulder blades. I glanced behind me and noticed that my new assistant was laughing uncontrollably. Confused, I wondered why he thought a shove was funny.

I soon realized that it was the newborn calf. Looking back over my shoulder I noticed that the persistent calf was standing behind me and giving me a look that had an unmistaken message, "Get out of my way, Doc."

After Larry controlled his laughter, he gently moved the calf back away from me and the mother cow. I went back to the process of completing the final skin sutures, and a few minutes later it was my turn to laugh as I noticed how the calf was wearing out my assistant as it was not going to take no for an answer.

I am happy to report that I was able to finish shortly thereafter and decided to let the calf nurse even before we allowed the cow to get up. By this time, the calf knew exactly what he wanted and how to get it. That nursing reflex I had felt earlier inside the uterus was now in full effect and working well. The mother and baby soon were up and moving out of the pen into the adjacent pasture. As they went out the gate, the calf slung his head in my direction as if giving me one last look that seemed to say, "Just remember Doc, stay out of my way."

CHAPTER 5
THE MIRACLE OF LIFE ELEPHANT STYLE

THE MOST AMAZING event I was involved with at the elephant sanctuary was the privilege of the birth process. We had an extended time to prepare for the deliveries since they have the longest gestational period of any mammal with an average pregnancy lasting 650 days. One of the most important duties I had was to make sure that these pregnant mothers would deliver viable, healthy babies. I needed to anticipate any possible complications that might threaten the health of the baby or its mother.

In the wild the entire herd is very important to the health and viability of the newest members. In the sanctuary the herd dynamic is different, but still was capably used to help teach the mother how to successfully deliver and raise a newborn. The other elephants as well as the sanctuary personnel are all considered part of the herd.

The Riddles and I took advantage of the lengthy pregnancy to make certain we had all the equipment needed and necessary medications readily available if there were any problems. We had oxygen in case the baby became hypoxic during or after the delivery. I had consulted with several experts who advised me on medications that might be needed. In the days and weeks before delivery we double-checked our prep and supplies list. The best part of the deliveries that I experienced was that none of the emergency medications were ever needed.

It was also important that we allowed

the other females in the herd to see and participate in the process of the delivery. In the wild the older females act like aunties, helping the new mother learn how to care for her new responsibility. The riddles took every opportunity to recreate this environment as best they could. I was extremely blessed to be a part of this process, and I was very lucky to be able to share this amazing experience with both of my young daughters.

After the baby was born and we determined it to be healthy, we made sure to give the mother and baby time to bond. Those first few moments are very important to develop that attachment that would be vital to the health and well-being of the newborn.

All the deliveries were different, but the one constant was the beautiful but over-sized babies. The weight of these newborns are an amazing 200 to 260 pounds. They can stand very soon after birth. In the wild it is very important for their safety so that they can become mobile quickly in order to survive. All baby animals I have been around are very cute, but I was always overwhelmed at how amazing newborn elephants are. Other than their size, the coolest feature is their active and expressive miniature trunks. This appendage has many different functions.

It is a nose with two nostrils and can be used like an arm with Asian elephants having one finger like tip at the end whereas African elephants have two. They use their trunks to pick up any number of large or small objects. They use it to suck up volumes of water and then to "blow" the water back into their mouth before swallowing. In those first few days the baby uses their trunk to explore its environment by smell and touch. As the baby would smell and caress my face with its delicate trunk, I would always feel an extremely strong emotional attachment to this amazing creature. The feeling of a strong bond has never been duplicated with any other animal over the course of my veterinary practice.

I consider the many years I was involved with the elephants to have provided me with some of the most memorable experiences of my career. Not many veterinarians get the opportunity to spend quality time with these incredible mammals and their dedicated caretakers.

CHAPTER 6

IT'S OKAY, IT COMES OFF ALL THE TIME

MY PRACTICE IS LOCATED in the central part of the state with the cities of Conway and Little Rock to the south and the Ozark Mountains to the north. Because of the location, my clientele is very diverse. Many are part of the growing group of professional ladies and gentlemen that work primarily in the cities. There are also many clients that are country folks, and their attitudes and language can be the source of some of the more interesting and funny encounters we have experienced.

One of these rural ladies was a 60 plus

year-old gray-haired woman who can be best described as having a demeanor that is a combination of sweetness, confidence, and being rough around the edges. Her name was Maggie Johnson, but she told us to call her Miss Maggie, and like most things she asked for, we did as she asked. She usually wore country style dresses and conservative black shoes. She walked with a distinctive limp, and her presence took over a room when she entered. Some folks that you can describe this way may come across as egotistical, but that is a word that you would never use when describing Miss Maggie.

One of the more memorable stories involving Miss Maggie came on her first visit to the clinic with her beloved male Collie dog named JJ. I was sitting in my office when I first heard her distinctive country drawl. A few minutes later Cathy, one of my vet assistants, came into my office with a big grin on her face to tell me that my appointment was ready to be seen.

I could tell that this new client had already worked her magic and charmed my employee. A few minutes later it seemed I had that same grin on my face. There was nothing that would be left unsaid if it crossed Miss Maggie's mind. After a few minutes of very entertaining chit-chat, I forced myself to start the exam of JJ.

The dog had been experiencing a variety of urinary tract symptoms that were described to us in great detail. Miss Maggie's interpretation of her dog straining to urinate also included colorful narrations of JJs' thoughts as he went through these difficulties. I did my best to hide my smile, but I noticed that Cathy was having more trouble as tears coursed down her cheeks and giggles took over her body. My physical examination of JJ turned up no specific conclusions or causes for his discomfort, so I decided that we needed to get to work and try to collect a urine sample. Cathy, JJ, Miss Maggie, and I all headed outside.

Cathy walked JJ to the grassy area beside the clinic, and I followed close behind with a long-handled plastic cup that we used to collect urine samples. It was soon evident that JJ had no interest in giving us a sample on demand. Miss Maggie watched us for a minute, then limped up to me, took my sample cup, grabbed the leash from Cathy and said, "Y'all move away. I'll show you how this is done."

Our grassy area has a slightly steep hill, and she quickly headed up the slope. Just about the time she reached the top, JJ decided to loop around Miss Maggie and head back to the bottom of the hill. The leash encircled her left leg, and I watched with mild panic as Miss Maggie fell to the ground with JJ tugging at the other end. It was then that the scene went from bad to completely surreal.

As I stood at the base of the hill in stunned shock as the leash yanked Miss Maggie's leg off her body. It then rolled down the hill. All I could see was her other leg sticking straight up in the air and her red plaid dress covering her head and shoulders. I should have immediately run up to assist her. I could not make my body move. It was then I noticed Cathy stood beside me, her mouth open and her eyes wide with shock.

About this time Miss Maggie rolled back to an upright sitting position, and JJ noticed his owners' distress. He did what Kathy and I should have done. As JJ walked back up the hill, Miss Maggie's' leg followed. As the collie reached her, she picked up the leg. It was a rough looking prosthetic with a black shoe attached. She replaced the leg in its proper position and then looked up at us. Noticing the stunned look on our faces, she jumped up with surprising ease and with only the slightest hint of embarrassment, declared loudly, "It's okay. It comes off all the time. "

Miss Maggie grabbed the leash and continued back up the hill to finish the process of getting a urine sample. Only then did my sense of chivalry come back to me. I quickly turned and walked up the hill to help. She gave me a wide smile but put her hand out in the standard stop signal and told me she had it under control. I did not argue and stopped in my tracks.

We watched as she picked up the cup and walked JJ around and soon collected the required specimen. Cathy took the sample and escaped inside. As Miss Maggie, JJ, and I walked back to the clinic she admitted that she needed to get a "new leg" since the old one came off too easily and often. I think she was more embarrassed about exposing herself and her underwear to this young vet than the leg coming off. It was good that the urine sample confirmed that JJ had a urinary tract infection and should be an easy treatment with some oral antibiotics. I don't think I could have handled any additional difficult diagnostics after that experience.

Miss Maggie and I continued to have a very good relationship over the years. Every once in a while, she would laughingly tease me about that first clinic visit. She may not have been considered a refined woman, but I always considered her a special lady and friend. I never asked her how she had lost her leg, and she never told me. She eventually moved to live with her daughter in California. I'll bet there are some good stories of her mixing with some of those California folks, but I'd be surprised if they were as good as the one about our first introduction.

CHAPTER 7

A FRIGHTENING EXPOSURE TO RABIES

AS VETERINARIANS we get used to treating life and death situations in animals but when we must deal with threats to our own health and the health of our own staff it takes on a high level of urgency. It started out as a routine appointment, although that was probably the only routine thing about this case.

It was a weekday afternoon in early July, when I invited a young woman with her one-year-old male pit bull into the exam room. The first unusual thing about the case was that six other young men and women followed the young lady and they all attempted to crowd into our small exam room. I couldn't help but notice the multiple tattoos and piercings. It was an interesting group, however I had to limit the numbers in the room to just three and I asked the rest to return to the front waiting room.

The presenting complaint for the young dog was that he had been having miscellaneous gastro-intestinal issues. The history given by the owner was vague and varied. I was not sure what I was going to find on exam. Wanda was my assistant on this day, and as was normal she proceeded me into the room and was gently holding the dog. When I first approach my patient, I always assess the attitude of the animal and place my hand up in greeting. I usually let the dog smell the back side of my hand in a non-threatening motion.

I followed this procedure with this young dog and noted that the dog did not show any overtly aggressive actions in my initial introduction, but as I attempted to pet him, he had placed its open mouth over my hand in a slightly strange manor. Since this action was a little unusual, and since it was a pit bull, I asked the owner if he had any previous aggression issues.

She seemed a bit indignant as she told me “No, it’s never bit anyone”.

I spent a few extra moments with the dog but had no further problems on my initial exam. Leaving the exam room for a moment, I found my stethoscope so I could complete my physical. As I returned, I once again placed my hand out in greeting. This was when everything suddenly changed for the worse.

The dog immediately and without hesitation bit my left hand as hard as it could. There had been no warning, and I was quite shocked by the new turn of events. The other thing that immediately got my attention was that he refused to let go. In an exam room full of people, no one seemed to notice that the dog had half my hand clamped tightly in that powerful jaw.

After what seemed like forever, but was probably only a couple seconds, I yelled. Unfortunately, my language was a bit harsher than usual. Wanda jumped into action and attempted to pry open his mouth. Pit Bulls have one of the strongest set of jaw muscles of any breed of dogs, and she could not get it to let go. By this time my office manager, Donna, also tried to come to my assistance, but she too was unable to free me. The young lady and her friends had done nothing up to this point to free my hand.

Finally, the dog's owner used two fingers to tap the dog firmly between the eyes. This tap got his attention, and he released me. I immediately ran out of the exam room to assess my physical condition as well as to get control of my emotions.

The bite had penetrated deep into both sides of my hand and the puncture site was bleeding a fair amount. Donna helped me to clean the wounds and to wrap my hand. I was able to collect myself and went back into the exam room.

The scene was actually peaceful, considering the turmoil I felt inside. The dog was calmly lying on the table with the owner holding him. Wanda was standing to the side, monitoring the dog but correctly keeping her distance.

Now that the dog had bitten a person there were several things I had to find out. First and most importantly I needed to know if the dog had been vaccinated for rabies by a veterinarian as required by state law. I had already looked at our record and I knew I had not done so at my clinic. I was disappointed but not surprised when the owner told me that she had not done the required vaccinations. We now had two problems. A sick dog and a possible rabies exposure to myself and to two of my staff.

Although none of my employees had been bitten, they had been exposed to the saliva. I decided to take the dog to a pen in the back while I questioned the owners more closely. I knew that this dog was just not acting normally, and I doubted if this was the first time it had acted like this. I asked the owner again if she was sure that the dog had never bitten anyone before. I noticed a suspicious glance exchanged between the owner and her friend. After a few moments they admitted that it had "playfully bitten a time or two before".

Keeping the dialogue open, I kept asking questions as their story kept changing, and soon determined that they were lying. I discovered that the incidents were worse and more numerous than they had admitted at first. I was in the middle of what was turning out to be more like an interrogation, when Wanda interrupted me and insisted that I immediately come to the back of the clinic.

As I went to the back of my clinic where the dog had been put into a cage, Wanda related her concerns on how he was acting "completely weird". At first the scene looked normal. The dog lay quietly at the back of the cage. As I walked closer and my foot was close to the small space just below the cage door, the dog suddenly charged and tried to attack. It kept trying to rip the wire of the cage for several seconds and suddenly calmed, appearing as though he was falling asleep again. I knew now we had big problems. This dog had severe neurologic issues and there was no way that I was going to put further staff at risk by trying to quarantine this dog for the required ten days. Rabies symptoms can be extremely variable, but symptoms such as what we were seeing made it very likely.

I knew that this was going to be a difficult conversation with the owner. As I returned to the exam room, I noticed that the attitude of her and her friends had deteriorated. They were obviously agitated and defensive. I explained what I had just seen with her dogs' neurologic disorders. I informed them that by law I was required by the State of Arkansas to report possible cases of rabies to the Health Department.

The response came from one of her friends who cussed me and demanded we must return the dog at once. Several more from her group heard the commotion and left the waiting room. This was when I knew I had to calm things down quickly. I told the owner that I needed to talk to her privately, finally agreeing that she could bring just one friend with her. Thankfully she chose a young man this time and not the woman who had become so irate. While the others filed out and made their way back to the waiting area, my office manager took me to the side to inform me that she had heard them talking. At least four other people had been previously bitten and that two young children had been at home with the dog.

With the owner's attention, I slowly and methodically explained the public health concerns that I had. I also explained the possible risk that the dog presented to her young children. I explained that unfortunately the only option I could see was to euthanize the dog and have the brain sent to the health department to have it tested for rabies. I told her that I did not see any other reasonable course of action. The only other option was to call in the sheriff and let the officers decide.

Upon my mentioning this option, they finally admitted that the sheriff had already been called on one of the previous bites and they had no interest in involving law enforcement again. As the story kept growing, I was becoming genuinely upset that the owner had lied to me about the previous biting incidents, but I did understand how difficult this decision was. She eventually went against the advice of several of her friends and decided to have her dog euthanized and consented to have the tests performed.

We carefully did the needed procedures so that no one else was exposed and we were able to do it efficiently and humanely. The samples were sent the next day to the State Health Department located in Little Rock. Several days later I was at home when my phone rang. The caller identified herself as the head doctor at Arkansas Health Department. When I heard her identify herself, I knew the news was not good. She told me that the dog had indeed tested positive for rabies. This meant that I had definitely been exposed as had any staff that had come into contact with the dogs' saliva which is where the virus is located in a rabid animal.

We spent the next thirty minutes on the phone as I reviewed all the information I knew about the case and the other known exposures that I had learned about. Unfortunately, because there were multiple exposures, all would need to get the prophylactic vaccinations as soon as possible at the hospital. The number and types of shots that would be needed would be different depending on a variety of factors. The good news was that the vaccinations were not as painful or have as many side effects as had been normal years ago. The other fact was that since we had correctly diagnosed this condition, no one would contract this deadly disease as long as everyone received the recommended treatments. We never found out how or when the dog had been exposed.

I was so thankful to my staff for their professionalism during this scary episode. I found out later that my rabies titers taken after the exposure confirmed that I likely had been exposed to active virus and that only proper administration of the pre- and post-exposure vaccinations had prevented me from getting this 99.9% fatal infection.

My staff and all the others that had been exposed were also effectively treated. Thank You, Lord.

CHAPTER 8
DIAGNOSIS: RINGWORM

AFTER MANY YEARS IN PRACTICE, I have learned one absolute truth about people in general and veterinary clients in particular. If you think you can predict what people are going to do or say, you will be proven wrong. Very wrong.

The interaction I have with my wonderful clients has always been a very major part of what I Love about being a veterinarian. As with many professions I have found that the majority of conversations with clients follow a predictable pattern, but every once in a while, I have been completely shocked. Take for example the case involving a simple ring worm.

Dermatology is the study of skin and problems with skin are common in dogs and cats. This has always been a very significant and important part of veterinary practice. Many times, skin problems are mentioned to me as an afterthought after doing other routine procedures. This was the case a few years back. I had just finished vaccinating a medium sized poodle for a middle-aged woman that had been in the clinic a few times before. As part of the process, I had done a routine exam and had not found any problems with this very pleasant dog. My normal procedure after finishing my examination is to ask the clients if there was anything else I could do for them. It is my experience that clients can sometimes delay their most important questions or comments till the very end of the exam time.

This was the case with this lady on this particular day. She suddenly had a very concerned look on her face and then asked me if her dog had a ringworm. Ringworm is a contagious skin problem in dogs that actually had nothing to do with worms. It was given this common name because the lesions often looked like a circular area of hair loss with the outer area having a red ring around it. I suspect that years ago before the cause of the lesions was known, people suspected a worm as the problem. It is now known that it is caused by a fungal infection of the skin. The disease can be passed between any animals as well as to humans and also can pass between people as well.

I was a little taken back by the question as was JoAnn, my vet assistant on this day. I had not seen any skin issues earlier but decided to do a second more detailed exam. After I was done with the second exam, I informed the dog's owner that I could not find any skin issues anywhere on the dog. I told her that ringworm could be difficult to diagnose in some cases, but that in this case I did not think her dog was infected.

She gave me a look of disbelief and stated that it had to have a ringworm. It was at this moment that I asked the question that caused the situation to go off the rails. "Why are you so sure your dog had ringworm."

She gave me a bit of a smirk. But instead of answering my question she quickly grabbed the bottom of her T-shirt and lifted it up above her naked breasts. She lifted her right breast up and asked, "Is this Ringworm?"

I did in fact see a classic ringworm lesion, and even though I tried, I could not answer her question. I could not speak. I could not even move for a moment or two. When I finally was able to make the connection from my brain to my body, I looked away and turned my attention to my assistant JoAnn. She also had a shocked expression, but she was at least able to respond. She gently moved between me and the client which broke the spell. I was finally able to speak and confirm her suspicions.

I explained that I was not allowed to diagnose human conditions, but did agree that the lesion did look like a ringworm. Only now did she lower her shirt and seem to understand that her display might have caused a sensation. I informed her that I could not tell her how she had gotten the lesion, but that I did not think it had come from her dog and that she needed to see her doctor for treatment. I then quickly left the room so that I did not get any further explanations or demonstrations.

As soon as the client left the clinic, JoAnn started giggling like a little girl and could not stop laughing for several long minutes. It was good that no other clients were there at the time, because we lost all pretense of professionalism over the next few moments. For several months after, my staff would ask me on occasion if I had diagnosed any ringworm lately, and then walk away laughing.

CHAPTER 9
EMPLOYEES ARE THE BACKBONE

HAVING a small business like a veterinary clinic for over 30-plus years means you have employed a very large number of men and women during that period of time. I am very proud of our history of keeping many employees for multiple years of dedicated service. We also have hired many young people that work for us during their high school and college years. Some have come to work thinking of a veterinary job as a place to love on animals and don't realize how hard the job can be. The diversity of my employees over the years has been amazing. Grandmas to teenagers- men and women (mostly women)-no experience to veterinary veterans. With only a few exceptions I have felt almost all of them have brought something positive to our clinic.

The employee that stands out to me was at the beginning of my career my boss. Her name was Judy, and she was Dr. McFarlin's' office manager when I was hired in the late 1980's. It was evident early on that she was my day-to-day supervisor. She considered the clinic to be her domain and she tolerated the veterinarians including her boss as a necessary part needed to provide care to the clients and animals. Over the two to three years that she was my supervisor we became good friends and trusted teammates. With that being said, she and I both knew she was in charge.

Judy was a middle-aged mother of two that had lived in the area around Greenbrier her entire life. I believe Judy knew almost everyone and if she did not know you or your family, she knew at least one of your friends. She was strong-willed and was willing to give you her opinion if asked and occasionally if she wasn't. All that strong attitude was wrapped up in one of the most loving and caring people I have ever met. If you or your animal were in need, she was definitely someone you wanted on your side.

She was on my side from the start, and she wanted to make sure my career and my life went well. She even tried to help this single young man find a good Christian woman to be my partner. This effort was not always appreciated by me as much as she would have liked. Approximately three years after being hired I negotiated to buy the clinic. Judy was very happy for me, but did not seem able to understand that this now made me the boss instead of her. She would allow me the right to act like the boss, but she just kept running the clinic like always. At first this bothered me a bit, then I decided that I would never find anyone that would work harder than she would to make my (her) clinic successful. Over time we were able to work together as a team and come to grips with the new reality- She Was Still the Boss.

I met my wife Kathy in January 1991, and our romance quickly progressed through the spring and summer. Judy did not introduce us, but she met her early on and was happy that I had found such a special person. The clinic usually did something special for my birthday and Kathy, Judy, and another employee named Sue worked together to celebrate it. I should have known that the three of them would hatch up some plan to give me some grief on my milestone 30th birthday. I showed up at Kathy's house for the party to find all my office staff plus their families gathered together. There was a very large cake sitting in the middle of the kitchen table. It looked like a big green hill with white footsteps going up one side and over the top. It said – UP-UP-AND-OVER-THE-HILL. They sang Happy Birthday and handed me the knife and told me to cut the cake. Someone in the back of the room yelled out-"Kill the Cake." I thought I would play along, so to the whole groups' chants of Kill the Cake; I turned the knife into a stabbing motion and plunged it deep into the top of the cake. Just before I did so I failed to notice that everyone had stepped back away from the cake. All I knew was that suddenly the large cake was Gone. Actually, more accurately the icing and wording was running off the table onto the floor. I had just "killed" a water balloon cake.

As the room erupted into laughter, I stood there with a blank look on my face. Only after I noticed that water and the icing were running off the table and into my shoes did I start to figure out what happened. By "killing the cake" I could not have done my part better even if I had been in on the joke. As it was, I was the target of one of the best birthday jokes ever. When I have a birthday cake that I'm cutting Kathy will occasionally give me a wry smile and ask if I want to "KILL the Cake."

Everyone who has owned and operated a small business knows that the employees are the backbone and the lifeblood of the organization. My business is no different. All the good veterinary medicine in the world will not keep clients happy if the staff is not doing a good job of supporting the clients and their animals. The clinic has been fortunate to have great employees over the years. Their hard work provides a reward for those of us who have been fortunate to spend our working days with animals and with the people who love them.

CHAPTER 10
FAMILY

THE FAMILY of a veterinarian is key to the success or potential failure of his or her career. This may be truer for veterinarians than many other professions due to the interaction the family has with the practice as well as the stresses that are placed on those we love.

Almost every small city or rural veterinary practice has had at least one if not all family members playing some role in the clinic. Over the years both of my children have worked for me for extended periods. My wife has worked in an advisory role off and on over the years when I needed it. This can be a source of great joy and family pride as well as stress and division. I am proud to say that we worked hard to keep our experiences as positive as possible over the years.

Certainly, one of the major stresses to a veterinarian's family is the demand of long hours. This was most evident early in my career when I was doing a great deal of large animal work and having to deal with a significant number of veterinary emergencies.

The phone rang one fall Saturday afternoon less than thirty minutes after I got home from the clinic. We opened every Saturday morning, but this Saturday was special. My wife and daughters were looking forward to a trip to the lake to go boating that afternoon. We had missed a trip the week previous when I got called in to work on my day off. I remember the looks on their faces. As soon as the phone rang both of my girls, now age ten and twelve, looked at me with disbelief and then frustration bordering on anger. They knew, just as I did, that this was probably another emergency call and that I couldn't ignore the call. It was important that I provided emergency services for my clients, and I had always tried my best to be there for them, but it exacted a toll on the relationship between me and my girls.

As I walked toward the phone, I felt a familiar knot in my stomach knowing our plans might be postponed once again. I had disappointed my eldest when I missed her soccer game last week and it was less than two weeks ago when I missed a game night with the family that my youngest was still mad at me about

As I answered the phone, perhaps my tone was a bit more unpleasant than I had meant for it to be. The caller identified himself as a veterinarian that worked for a large circus. As I realized he was not one of my normal clients, I began to feel mildly optimistic about our plans for the afternoon. It was not long into the conversation though that my hopes were dashed.

The circus was in Little Rock, about a forty-five-minute drive from Greenbrier. They had an elephant that was part of their show that needed attention as soon as possible. They had no way to get one of their attending veterinarians to Little Rock in time and they were looking for help. I made the decision that they would need to find someone else to help them out. I would have to be gone all afternoon for such a call, and I decided that I was not going to disappoint my girls again. I explained the situation and he said he understood.

We continued to get ready for our boat trip, and then the phone rang again. The same veterinarian said that he knew I had experience with elephants, and they really needed my services. I decided to stand my ground this time and keep the promise I had made to the girls but before I could reply he proposed a deal that included my family too. He would provide backstage passes for the entire family to see all the animals before the circus performance as well as free tickets to the show. I would have to give up another Saturday afternoon to work, but it would be more than worth it to provide this opportunity to my wife and daughters. Maybe the boat ride could wait. I asked him to hold on a moment while I asked the girls. It did not take more than a second for their response of shouts with excitement, “We’re going to the circus! Yeaaaaaa!”

I was the hero.

From what I could determine, the elephant I was going to see had a likely intestinal impaction causing abdominal pain. This same condition in horses is called colic and it is treated in a similar way.

After arriving at the circus location and finding the woman in charge of the elephants, we were led to a large Asian female named JoJo. As I began to prepare to treat her, a good-looking young man appeared. He was assigned to escort my family for a full backstage tour of any of the animals they wanted to see. By the joy on their faces, the frustration of their dad's profession and a day on the lake were quickly forgotten as they happily walked away. I was left to the task of treating JoJo.

In assessing my patient, I learned that she had not eaten for 24 hours and was showing some mild symptoms of abdominal pain. Thankfully elephants are not as debilitated by the pain as horses when they colic, but it is still very important that I would quickly relieve the pain and the intestinal impaction that was most likely the cause.

After questioning the caretaker further, I found that JoJo had been housed at her last location on a sandy bed. I suspected that she might have eaten sand and that this had caused the problem. Treatment for colic for JoJo the elephant is basically the same as for horses. We would give pain meds to relax her and her intestinal tract. I was able to give an intramuscular injection of pain meds that worked quickly to calm her. My next course of action was to attempt to get mineral oil into intestines.

This might be a bit more challenging. In horses we use a long tube inserted through the nose and into the stomach. Since elephants have a very sensitive and long trunk, I would not be able to give it in that way. This is where I was hoping that the very good training these magnificent animals received would allow us to give the mineral oil orally.

The training and care of all the animals at this particularly large circus was second to none. The trainer was able to encourage JoJo to swallow a gallon of mineral oil by slowly giving it to her by mouth. You could tell she did not like the consistency or taste of the oil, but she trusted her trainer and was willing to drink it.

We then decided that a gallon of oil should be given twice more over the next twelve hours. I also dispensed more pain medication to be given if needed. Within thirty minutes JoJo had drank some water and started eating some hay. She no longer showed any signs of pain or abdominal discomfort. As I finished the examination, she placed her trunk on the top of my head and took in a deep breath. The trainer laughed as she told me that my smell would always be remembered by this very smart creature.

I hoped that the memories were mostly positive. I decided it was safe to leave her to rest for the afternoon and evening. I would check her again later that night. She would be given several days to rest before she would rejoin the nightly performance.

I met up with my wife and girls just as they finished their tour. They could not stop chattering about all the amazing animals they had seen. Both daughters gave me an impromptu hug. I was a happy dad.

The circus treated us to a free dinner backstage with the crew. We listened to many interesting stories about the animals and the amazing team that cared for them on a regular basis. After eating it was time to find our seats for the show as the crew went to dress for their parts. The circus was a three-ring extravaganza that held us all captivated. It was made even more special as the girls would yell out the names of the particular animals as they came into the arena, and they were able to tell me little tidbits about them.

After the show we made our way to

the backstage area where I was happy to see that JoJo was doing very well. She had just finished her second dose of mineral oil and was happily eating some more hay. Once again as I examined her, she smelled of my head and then went back to eating with a contented moan. I could not have been paid a higher compliment.

As we drove back home with two tired but contented girls, I thought to myself how lucky I was. Despite the long hours and demand on my time, I felt blessed to be able to work in a profession where I had the ability to share some of my most amazing experiences with my family. Their love and support over the years means everything to me.

AUTHOR NOTES

After working over 30 years in Arkansas as a small and large animal veterinarian has generated many amazing memories. As I think back about my life to this point it is my belief that relationships are the most important part of any person's career. This is especially true for veterinarians. We have the opportunity to create and develop relationships with amazing animals, dedicated owners, and our talented staff. Emotions are a regular component of my daily experience on any given day. They can involve joy, amazement, sadness, gratitude, and of course humor.

As I begin the process of telling stories involving my career, I have to start with the history that made me the person I am today. My family is full of medical experience, so it is no surprise that I ended up as a veterinarian. As I grew up, I was surrounded with an amazing group of nurses. My mother had the most influence on me as a nurse, but I also had two aunts, a grandmother, and two other extended family that chose this noble profession. I learned about dedication and caring for your patients from this group of talented women. I also had several relatives involved as farmers, livestock producers, and other professionals that taught me about commitment and hard work. The profession of veterinary medicine was represented to me by my father in a manner that I do not believe could have been exceeded.

After graduating from Colorado State University Veterinary School, he was offered a job in a mixed small and large animal practice in New Zealand. There was a need for veterinarians for many of the rural practices in this small country, so the government was willing to subsidize our family's move. My Dad was a hard worker and fit in well with these genuine people with their English heritage. He never knew from day to day if he would be working with dogs, cats, cattle, pigs, horses, or sheep. He later taught me this ability to be flexible and adjust to multiple challenges. I was three years old when we moved, and we stayed there for three years. The pastures were green, and the hills were dotted with many white sheep. It was a good place for a young kid to grow up, learning about a variety of farm animals.

We then lived in Australia for a year, and I got even more diverse experiences in this vast and amazing country before moving back to the U.S. when I was seven years old. We lived in Colorado again for three years as my father went back to school for his master's degree before moving to Arizona to work for a large feedlot as a resident veterinarian. After five years there, we then moved to Texas where my father was hired to work for a veterinary pharmaceutical company. Living in multiple locations and observing the many facets of the veterinary profession were very important in developing my flexibility as a person and as a veterinarian. I felt I could live anywhere and learn to adjust to all types of people and locations.

The Texas Panhandle was where I went to high school and completed my first four years of college. I graduated with a degree in animal science and then was accepted into veterinary school at Texas A&M University. Those four years were some of the toughest, but also the most rewarding years of my life. I learned about all the amazing details of the animals I had been around. As I began looking for my first job, I decided to try to find one in a mixed practice doing small and large animal medicine.

I found just such a job. I began my career as an associate veterinarian at the practice that I later owned in Greenbrier, Arkansas. I worked for a very talented and hardworking boss named Dr. Bob McFarland. He was interested in specializing in racehorse medicine and he was counting on me to keep the thriving practice going strong while he explored this new interest. The community welcomed me, and I eventually purchased the clinic as Bob went on to start a new racetrack equine practice.

Four years after moving to Greenbrier I met and married the most amazing woman I had ever met. She continues to this day to be my motivation and my lifetime love. We have been blessed with two beautiful and very talented daughters. My family and I have embraced this community, and it has done likewise to us. The practice has changed and grown over the years as we moved from mixed large and small animal to exclusively small animal during the last few years of operation.

The chapters that follow are a collection of stories told to show the relationships and emotions that have made up my practice over these past 30 plus years. They are based on true stories, although I have changed some minor details as well as many of the names of staff, clients, and animals. I hope you enjoy reading this collection.

Thank you for trusting me with care of your animals,

Carl Fulton, DVM

ABOUT THE AUTHOR

Carl Fulton, DVM, practiced in Greenbrier, Arkansas, operating Faulkner County Veterinary Clinic for thirty-five years. Dr. Fulton obtained a bachelor's degree in animal science from West Texas State University and completed his Doctor of Veterinary Medicine at Texas A&M College Station. His practice in Greenbrier included small pets as well as livestock and elephants. He and his wife Kathy have two daughters. He has loved the years that he practiced veterinary medicine and the stories he got from his experiences.

Made in the USA
Monee, IL
04 November 2026

67375580R00066